Y0-EHG-303

Sleep Apnea

The Ultimate Guide How To Manage And Treat Your Sleep Apnea

Table Of Contents

Introduction

I want to thank you and congratulate you for buying the book, *Sleep Apnea: The Ultimate Guide How To Manage And Treat Your Sleep Apnea.*

This book contains proven steps and strategies on how to manage Sleep apnea by using conventional and alternative therapies.

Many people experience sleep disturbance, not knowing the cause and how to manage it. Some of these sleep disturbances are caused by stress, certain physical activities and by intake of medicines and other substances that can alter sleep patterns. But aside from these factors, some sleep disturbances are caused by a real pathologic disorder- which may stem from either a defect of the structures of the brain or in the signaling mechanisms involving the respiratory organs.

Recognition and treatment of sleep disorders are vital to one's health to prevent complications. One sleep disorder that can greatly affect the quality of one's life is sleep apnea. Different treatment modalities of this condition are now being used and this book will give you some tips on how to manage your sleep apnea.

Thanks again for buying this book. I hope you enjoy it!

Chapter 1 Introduction to Sleep Apnea

Sleep is one of the basic needs of a man. Experts say that people need 6 to 7 hours of sleep for optimum functioning throughout the day. A recent study shows that lack of sleep is even more fatal than lack of food and water. The latter can kill you in a month, while the former can kill you in 11 days.

People encounter different sleeping experiences per day. Most people would normally have a good night's sleep with dreams in between, but some would encounter sleeping problems, like difficulty going to sleep or insomnia, difficulty of going back to sleep after waking up in the middle of the night, while some would have nightmares that wake them up from their sleep. These conditions can lead to a sleep pattern disturbance that can eventually progress to a sleeping disorder.

One of these sleeping disorders, and possibly, one of the most undiagnosed conditions, is sleep apnea, which can either be central, obstructive (OSA) or mixed. Sleep apnea is a condition characterized by a disturbance of sleep caused by cessation of breathing. Gaps in respiration may last for more than 10 seconds and can occur several times during a 7-hour sleep period. Have you ever experienced suddenly waking up in the middle of the night trying to catch your breath as if you have been strangled? You may think that this is due to a nightmare, but it is actually caused by pauses in respiration. Snoring is actually one of its manifestations. The sound that is produced when you snore is the result of a compensatory mechanism of the body to catch your breath.

Sleep apnea can be caused by different factors. Studies show that obesity is significantly linked to the development of OSA. The accumulation of fat in the abdomen can compress the diaphragm and impede its expansion during breathing or fat can also accumulate in the air passages, blocking the entry of air into the lungs. These then decrease the depth and rate of respiration, causing apnea.

Central sleep apnea, on the other hand, is caused by a defect in the respiratory centers in the brain. The respiratory centers, namely the medulla and pons, regulate and control the respiratory cycle. Any disturbance in the functioning of these two neurologic structures, or in the signaling pathways to and from these structures, can suppress the respiratory drive of a person. In contrast to what the most of people think, oxygen is not the major driver of respiration but the level of carbon dioxide. An increase in carbon dioxide levels signals the brain to stimulate the respiratory structures in order to eliminate this gaseous material. Therefore, any alteration in the signaling pathway or in the feedback mechanism between the brain and respiratory structures can cause an apnea.

Smoking is also associated with sleep apnea. A stick of cigarette contains 4000 toxic chemicals that can alter the different functions of the body. One of these toxic chemicals is nicotine, which relaxes the respiratory muscles in the chest. Relaxation of these muscles decreases the expansion and movement of the lungs, thus decreasing the amount of air entering the airway.

Any structural abnormality that involves the upper and lower airways can cause respiratory depression and apnea. Obstruction of the nasal passages, which may be due to common cold, deviation of the nasal septum, or a tumour can promote sleep apnea.

Many people experiencing sleep apnea don't recognize that they have the sleeping disorder. This may inadvertently go on for years without diagnosis. Some patients may also be immune to the side effects of lack of sleep, such as fatigue and irritability. These people may or may not experience symptoms unless they wake up in the middle of the night due to lack of air or someone else tell them that they are snoring or choking. Other symptoms of this condition are associated with the effects of lack of sleep the following day. These include inability to concentrate, impairment of memory and headaches.

Sleep apnea has been traditionally managed with CPAP or continuous positive airway pressure, a type of mechanical ventilation that assists the patient in breathing. But due to its interference with most activities of the patients during the day, a lot of treatment modalities have been introduced. These include Provent Therapy and complementary therapies like yoga and acupressure. Lifestyle modification also plays a role in managing sleep apnea. These treatment regimens are discussed in the succeeding chapters.

Chapter 2 The Conventional Therapies

The probability of developing more severe disorders in sleep apnea is high. A higher propensity for heart attack and stroke is attributed to sleep apnea and so do arrhythmias and hypertension. A continuous decrease in respiration and subsequently oxygen delivery to the tissues lead to hypoperfusion of vital organs, predominantly of the heart and of the brain. Thus, treatment of sleep apnea must be implemented right away to decrease these life-threatening complications.

Treatment of sleep apnea depends upon the severity of the disorder and the characteristics of the patient. For moderate to severe sleep apnea, most doctors recommend the patient to use CPAP. Since apnea occurs due to obstruction, narrowing and collapse of the airway, CPAP serves as a stent or splint to the respiratory passages to maintain their patency. It works by delivering positive pressure through a tubing that connects the facial mask to the flow generator. This then prevents the airways from collapsing. This mask has to be worn all throughout the sleeping period and most patients with moderate to severe apnea may require lifetime assistance by a CPAP machine.

Many studies have already shown the efficacy of this treatment modality. CPAP is shown to prevent wakefulness at night, improve neurologic symptoms like improved concentration and memory, and improved quality of life among patients with this condition. However, this treatment regimen is not shown to be effective in reducing respiratory difficulties among patients with mild sleep apnea.

CPAP, just like any medicines, has adverse effects that you should watch out for. Since CPAP makes use of a facial mask, most of its side effects are associated with nasal and paranasal problems. The delivery of air into the nasal passages can create friction to the mucosa of the nose and this may cause rhinitis. The shear force produced by the pressure generated by the machine, plus the drying effect of the cool air produced, cause inflammation of the nasal mucosa. Nasal sores can also occur as a result of the friction produced by the prolonged contact of the mask to the nasal bridge, especially if the mask is applied tightly. To prevent these adverse effects, you should set the flow generator to its proper settings. The concentration of oxygen should be set to the prescribed setting and the mask should be applied snugly. Abdominal bloating can also occur as a result of swallowed air.

Many patients do not like this treatment modality because it requires careful maintenance and adequate knowledge about the machine. Most patients, especially the older ones, are afraid of using these machines because of the technical knowledge that it requires. Most of the time, a private nurse is needed by these patients to help them with the use of CPAP.

More recently, an alternative treatment to CPAP had been introduced. They call it Provent therapy, which does not require a machine anymore. This device is applied orally to hold the structures in the mouth from prolapsing into the airway, especially the tongue. This device maintains airway patency during sleep.

Studies comparing the efficacy of CPAP and this oral device show that in mild to moderate sleep apnea, these two treatment modalities are both successful in preventing sleep apnea with equal levels of efficacy. In terms of quality of sleep, these two regimens also show the same level of success in enhancing sleep quality. An intra-oral device may also decrease the sleepiness of patients at daytime and decrease incidence of fatigability, anxiety and mood changes during the day. Patients also show to prefer this device over CPAP because of lesser discomfort and easy usage. Snoring may also be decreased with this intra-oral device.

In essence, Provent therapy can be used as an alternative treatment when patients cannot tolerate CPAP. However, just like CPAP, it has its own side effects. Short-term problems may include hypersalivation, or an increase in the saliva production during sleep. This is in response to the presence of a foreign body in the mouth which may stimulate the salivary glands to produce more saliva. Another short-term side effect is teeth discomfort. Since this intra-oral device serves like a brace, patients may feel pain in their teeth in the first few days of their use. Both hypersalivation and teeth discomfort are reduced with prolonged use of an intra-oral device.

The long-term side effects, on the other hand, may include dislodgement of the device, along with jaw discomfort. The intra-oral device must be regularly replaced to prevent complications like infection. Research shows that the use of an intra-oral device is cheaper than a CPAP machine. This is one of the reasons why patients choose this modality over CPAP.

Chapter 3 The Complementary Therapies

Yoga is one of the most famous alternative practices nowadays. Different illnesses or disorders have already been managed by this therapy and many people are now trying yoga out. Though yoga has been famous for its benefits in breathing, in relaxation and in keeping you physically fit, recent studies have shown that yoga can also be used in sleep disorders, such as sleep apnea.

The use of yoga in sleep apnea stems out from different factors. First, yoga can improve breathing. Since breathing is one of the main problems in sleep apnea, yoga can definitely prevent breathing problems during sleep. It enhances the delivery of oxygen to the tissues, most especially to the brain and heart, and can prevent the collapse of airways as it stimulates respiratory drive.

Second, yoga can be used as a weight loss regimen. It has already been mentioned that one of the risk factors for sleep apnea include obesity and so losing weight through yoga could be an effective way of decreasing incidence of sleep apnea. This effect, however, is not instant, as you would need multiple yoga sessions to lose weight.

Third, many experts say that sleep apnea can also be caused by imbalances in the different chemicals in the brain that are involved in sleep. One of these chemicals, also known as neurotransmitters, is serotonin. This neurotransmitter regulates the sleep-wake cycle and any alteration in the levels of this neurotransmitter can cause sleep disorders. Yoga can control the levels of this neurotransmitter, thus helping further in the improvement of sleep apnea.

Because of all these benefits that one can get from yoga, experts have devised some yoga exercises to prevent sleep apnea. These exercises are usually done before going to sleep. Here are some of their recommended exercises.

1. Deep breathing

You can do this exercise anywhere- on your bed, on the couch or on the floor, and you can do this either sitting or lying down. First, you must keep your spine straight and your shoulders relaxed. Put your right hand on your abdomen and slowly inhale deeply as you feel your abdomen expand. Hold your breath for 5 seconds and slowly exhale. During exhalation, try to push your belly in. Do this 10 times with 10 seconds rest in between.

2. Against the Wall

Lie down on the floor and position yourself perpendicular to a wall. Raise your legs up the wall until your hips touch the wall. Spread your arms on each side and keep your legs as far as you can. Slightly bend your knees to slightly relax your legs and abdomen. Do deep breathing, as indicated in the previous number, 10 times with eyes closed.

3. Pigeon-like Position

Sit on the floor with your right leg extended backwards and your left leg folded in front facing the right. Position your arms on both sides of your left leg while keeping your back straight. Place a pillow in front of your left leg and slowly bend forward as low as you can. Rest your chest and abdomen on the pillow while spreading your arms to your sides. Turn your head to whichever side you prefer. On this position, do deep breathing 5 times. Do the same thing with your left leg extended backward.

4. Cobra Position

Lie down on your stomach with your legs extended backward and your arms on your side but not spreading it laterally. Keep your palms flat close to your chest. As you inhale deeply, try to push your spine upward while slowly extending the neck up. Elbows should be extending as you lengthen your spine. Go as far as you can comfortably can but keep your shoulders relaxed. Exhale as you reach your farthest stretch and continue exhalation as you go back to your prone position. Do this 5 times with 8 seconds rest in between.

Another complementary therapy gaining popularity for the management of sleep apnea is auricular acupressure. The ears, as believed by the Chinese, contain different points corresponding to different parts or systems of the body. Points, such as Lung and Endocrine points, are located in the ears, which could be stimulated to improve symptoms of sleep apnea.

Pressing the acupressure lung point stimulates the respiratory muscles of the upper airways to keep them from collapsing during sleep. This effect is mediated by applying pressure on certain lung points in the ear to relieve the symptoms of sleep apnea. Studies show that acupressure can significantly lower the incidence of sleep apnea in contrast to patients who are not receiving acupressure. A limitation, however, of auricular acupressure is that it is not effective for severe sleep apnea.

Thus, the efficacy of acupressure depends on the severity of the condition. The efficacy decreases as severity of sleep apnea increases.

Some of the acupressure points, some are outside the ears, that are helpful for sleep apnea are Neiguan, Shenmen, Shimien and Anmien points.

1. Neiguan

Stimulation of Neiguan point promotes relaxation. This pressure point is not located in the ears, but on the wrist, instead. To locate this pressure point, place three fingers on the wrist with palms facing upward. Be sure that you are not pressing on the pulse because this will block perfusion to your hands. The Neiguan point is located on the central depression in between the tendons on your wrist. Press on this point intermittently before sleeping to make you feel relaxed.

2. Shenmen

The Shenmen point, which is also used in relieving addiction, is stimulated to regulate functions of the heart. This point is located in the inner fold of your auricle. Using your index finger, locate for the depression in your auricle just before the entrance to the external auditory canal. Press this for 20 seconds to have a good night's sleep.

3. Shimien

The Shimien point is most effective for insomnia but is also used for other sleep disorders. This is located on the sole of the foot. To locate it, draw an imaginary line at the center of the sole of the foot and between two ankle bones. Pressing the point of interaction of these two imaginary lines shouldn't be painful. Relief from sleeping difficulties results from pressing this point.

4. Anmien

Anmien point promotes peaceful sleep. This point is located right below the ear, at the bottom of your jaw. Using your index and middle finger, press this point until calmness seeps into you.

Chapter 4 Food Therapy

Eating is one of the most common stress-relieving factors being used by many people. Ice cream, chocolates, cakes and different comfort foods can all promote relief of anxiety and enhance the feeling of well-being. But aside from all of these benefits of eating, there are certain foods that can promote sleep and prevent sleep disorders, like sleep apnea. Experts say that diet can absolutely affect one's quality of sleep and reduce sleep apnea.

Sleep apnea does not just affect your quality of sleep, but can also affect your quality of life. Sleep disturbance caused by this condition can induce a variety of changes in your daily activities. Lack of sleep delivers less oxygen to the brain causing a decrease in the level of functioning of the brain. As mentioned in the previous chapters, lack of sleep can cause easy fatigability and impairment of neurologic functions. These neurologic symptoms can prevent you from functioning to your optimum and can consequently affect your job and personal life negatively.

To alleviate these symptoms of sleep apnea, a change in the foods you eat can be instituted. Most experts suggest a Mediterranean diet, a Greek- inspired diet composed of vegetables, fruits, nuts, oats and seafood. This diet is low in fats and sodium, which are increased in obesity and hypertension. The institution of this type of diet in sleep apnea rests on the principle that these foods can help control obesity, improve brain functioning, which can be altered in sleep apnea, and reduction of complications of this condition, such as heart attack and stroke.

A study in Greece showed that the incidence of sleep apnea among patients who took Mediterranean diet decreased compared to those who had no diet modification. Aside from the reduction in the incidence of sleep apnea, there were also associated health benefits shown with this diet. Patients who took Mediterranean diet lost weight, increased their physical activities and complied more to the diet program. This diet regimen had also shown a tremendous decrease in the incidence of sleep apnea complications like heart attack.

What foods can you eat to improve your sleep apnea? Here are some of them:

1. Fish Oil

Fish oils are rich in omega-3 fatty acids that are scientifically proven to decrease incidence of heart diseases. These fatty acids are associated with a decrease in the body's levels of low density lipoproteins, also known as bad cholesterol, because they distribute cholesterol to the tissues; and an increase in the levels of high-density lipoproteins, or good cholesterol, because they transport cholesterol from the cells to the liver for metabolism. The health benefits of fish oils and their effects on sleep apnea are attributed to the management of obesity. Omega- 3 fatty acids also have beneficial effects to the brain, thus relieving possible defects of signaling pathways associated with sleep apnea. Tuna, mackerel, sardines and salmon are rich in omega-3.

2. Fiber

A diet high in fiber and low in calorie can improve symptoms of sleep apnea because of their effects on weight and digestion. Weight loss promotes the removal of the excess fats on the abdomen, thus giving more space for the expansion of the diaphragm. This can also remove excess fats that may be obstructing your airway, thus keeping your lungs and other air passages patent. Fiber is found in fruits, vegetables, whole grains and oats.

Using all these foods to improve your sleep apnea, here is a simple recipe that can help you prepare a Mediterranean diet. This is called **Mediterranean Seafood Vegetable Salad.**

Ingredients:

- 1 can Tuna, flaked
- 1 can Salmon, flaked
- ¼ cup Mayonnaise
- Lettuce
- ¼ cup pineapple chunks
- 1 onion, sliced
- ¼ cup roasted nuts, chopped
- Olives

Procedure:

1. Drain tuna and salmon and mix everything in a bowl except lettuce and nuts.

2. Assemble the salad on a plate. Spread lettuce leaves on the plate first, followed by the fish mixture.

3. Top with chopped nuts and serve.

Chapter 5 The Oil Therapy

Different essential oils are now being used for different purposes. Though these essential oils are mostly used for relaxation and aromatherapy, a lot of essential oils are now used for specific disorders or illnesses. Some of these illnesses include infection, arthritis, toothache and constipation. Through continuous advocacy of the use of essential oils, their use has already included sleep disorders, like sleep apnea.

Essential oils are compounds that are extracted from plant parts, such as leaves, stems, flowers and roots. These essential oils emit an aromatic scent that is calming to nerves, which is one of its main uses. Essential oils also contain antioxidants and phytochemicals which can help in fighting different diseases, like cancer and cardiovascular diseases.

Some of the essential oils attributed to improvement of sleep apnea are lavender oil, sandalwood oil, valerian root oil and marjoram oil.

1. Lavender Oil

This oil is one of the most favourite essential oils in the world, being known for its aromatic scent and relaxing properties. Its oil comes from the flower of the lavender plant. One of its documented uses is its benefit in sleep disorders. Due to its vasodilating properties, or its ability to increase the size of the lumen of blood vessels, more oxygenated blood can go to the brain, thus can improve brain functions. If used before bedtime, lavender oil can promote quality of sleep because of its calming, relaxing and soothing effects. To use for sleep apnea, massage onto forehead and temple for a few minutes until calmness sets in.

2. Valerian Root Oil

One of the most famous effects of valerian root oil is its tranquilizing and sedating effects. It contains valerenic acid, which is beneficial to nervous system functioning. This effect reduces incidence of sleep pattern disturbance and can promote quality of sleep. It has also effects on the airways. They relax the airways, letting more air to enter the lungs. The application of this oil is similar to that of lavender oil. Just massage onto temple or forehead and you can expect a good night's sleep.

3. Chamomile Oil

Aside from the sweet aroma of chamomile, this oil promotes peaceful sleep. Extracted from the flower of chamomile plant, this oil contains antioxidants that help fight a variety of diseases and can help prevent complications of sleep apnea, such as heart attack and stroke. It can also relieve stress and anxiety which may aggravate the condition. The application is similar to that of the previous essential oils discussed.

4. Sandalwood Oil

One of the most remarkable components of Sandalwood oil is sisqueterpenes, a compound that can stimulate the pineal gland in the brain. This gland is known for its production of melatonin, which is also a sleep inducer. Stimulation of this gland promotes better and deeper sleep, calmness and clarity of the mind. This prevents wakefulness in the middle of the night and can promote better respiration. Sandalwood is also known to cause soothing of the limbic lobe, which is a part of the brain dedicated to emotions. Soothing of this part of the brain removes emotional stress, thus, promoting sleep.

5. Marjoram Oil

This oil helps in improving sleep apnea by preventing snoring. This oil, unlike the other four which are topically applied, is used via inhalation of its essence. Keeping the bottle of oil open, the essence of this oil promotes relaxation of the airway and relieves the obstruction present that can cause snoring and sleep apnea.

Chapter 6 The Natural Therapy

In any disease, natural therapy can help a lot. This therapy is mostly composed of lifestyle modifications, organic products and exercise routines that can relieve the symptoms of diseases. This therapy can be instituted to manage heart diseases, as well as sleeping disorders.

Sleep apnea, as discussed in the first chapter, can be caused and precipitated by a multitude of factors. Most of these factors are modifiable, like obesity and smoking. These modifiable factors will be the focus of the natural therapy.

Some exercises, like orofacial exercises, are said to be helpful in relieving sleep apnea. The main goal of these exercises is to strengthen the respiratory muscles and prevent them from relaxation. Noncompliance of these respiratory muscles can cause decreased expansion of lungs, thus causing shallow breathing. This type of breathing can lower the oxygen content of the blood and can subsequently cause sleep apnea. The orofacial parts that are worked out in these exercises are the tongue, the jaw, the throat, the soft palate and the face.

The tongue, though is one of the strongest muscles in the body, can also weaken due to a variety of reasons. Weakness of the tongue, plus the relaxing effect of sleep on the muscles, can cause prolapse of the tongue to the back of the throat, which can block your air passages. It is important to strengthen this muscle to prevent such life-threatening phenomenon.

The jaw also plays a role in keeping the airway patent. If jaw is too tensed, relaxation of the muscles supporting it would be impossible. Tightness of jaw muscles can prevent the jaw from opening during sleep, thus preventing entry and exit of air. This is most especially prominent when the patient has obstructive sleep apnea.

The throat and the soft palate also need to be strong in order to keep the airway open.

Collapse of the throat and flapping over of the soft palate can lead to a blocked airway.

Here are some of the orofacial exercises effective for sleep apnea.

1. Tongue Exercise

Tongue slide aims to strengthen your tongue muscles. To do this, place the tip of your tongue behind your upper front teeth. From this position, slowly move the tip of the tongue backward, following the contour of the soft palate, as far as you can. Do this with the mouth closed and open.

2. Throat Exercise

This exercise aims to strengthen the muscles of your throat. You may need a mirror in this exercise because you need to observe the movement of your uvula and tongue. To do this, open your mouth as wide as you can. Stick out your tongue, preferably downward, and observe your uvula in the mirror. The uvula, which is the structure at the center of the palate, should elevate as you stick your tongue out. Hold this position for 5 seconds and repeat 5 times.

3. Soft Palate Exercise

This exercise aims to strengthen the muscles of your soft palate and keep the pharynx open. The lungs are also being exercised in this activity. To do this, inhale slowly through your nose. Hold your breath for 3 to 5 seconds before exhaling. As you exhale, keep your lips pursed together, as if blowing a candle. Exhale for 5 seconds, keeping your lips pursed all the time. Repeat 5 times.

Aside from exercises, weight control and smoking cessation are keys to relieving sleep apnea. Weight control measures have already been included in the previous chapters. Smoking cessation may not be easy but you can ask for help from support groups or from your doctor. Good sleeping habits can also help you with promoting a good night's sleep and prevent symptoms of sleep apnea. Here are some tips on how to improve quality of sleep:

1. Lie on your side

Lying on your back can create an equal pressure between the upper and lower parts of your body. This can increase fluid flow into your lungs that can aggravate sleep apnea. Lying on one's side can alleviate this effect and improve your respiration during sleep.

2. Avoid caffeine or nicotine before sleeping

Caffeine and nicotine are both stimulants, which can hinder you from sleeping early. They can also cause spasm of airways, which can lead to difficulty of breathing. There is increased risk of sleep apnea with these agents. Foods rich in caffeine include chocolates, tea, soft drinks and coffee. Avoid sugar-rich foods as they can also increase energy supply, thus inhibiting you from going to sleep.

3. Eat light

Fullness can cause difficulty of breathing, especially at night. This can limit the expansion of diaphragm, thus augmenting sleep apnea. Eat light during dinner and avoid lying down right after eating.

Sleep apnea is caused by many factors, which can also be reversed by different treatment measures. CPAP and Intra-oral devices are devices that are used for moderate to severe apnea, while alternative and complementary modalities can be used as adjunct therapies in sleep apnea. Yoga, acupressure, orofacial exercises, essential oils, proper diet and good sleeping habits are all helpful in preventing sleep apnea and relieving its symptoms. It is important to recognize sleep apnea early to prevent its progression to fatal complications, like heart attack and stroke.

Conclusion

Thank you again for buying this book!

I hope this book was able to help you to understand sleep apnea and how to manage it.

The next step is to try these alternative therapies to manage your sleep apnea.

Finally, if you enjoyed this book, please take the time to share your thoughts and post a review on Amazon. It'd be greatly appreciated!